Book Title: "Metabolism Mastery: Breaking Free from Sabotaging Habits"...

Table of Contents...

Introduction: Understanding Metabolism...

Chapter 1: The Importance of Metabolism...

Chapter 2: Eating Habits and Their Impact on Metabolism...

Chapter 3: The Role of Physical Activity in Boosting Metabolism...

Chapter 4: Sleep and Stress - Unseen Factors Affecting Metabolism...

Chapter 5: Hydration and Its Influence on Metabolism...

Chapter 6: The Power of Nutrient Timing...

Chapter 7: Superfoods for Metabolic Health...

Chapter 8: Metabolism and Aging - What You Need to Know...

Chapter 9: Hormones and Metabolism - Balancing the Scales...

Chapter 10: Mindful Eating for a Revved-Up Metabolism...

Chapter 11: Building Lean Muscle Mass for Metabolic Efficiency...

Chapter 12: The Impact of Genetics on Metabolism...

Chapter 13: Supplements and Metabolism - Sorting Fact from Fiction...

Chapter 14: Lifestyle Changes for a Lasting Metabolic Transformation...

Chapter 15: Maintaining Your Metabolic Momentum...

Introduction: Understanding Metabolism...

Metabolism, often described as the body's engine, is a complex set of chemical reactions that occur within us every day, allowing us to breathe, think, and move. It plays a pivotal role in maintaining our overall health and well-being. Yet, many of us unknowingly engage in habits that sabotage our metabolism, leading to weight gain, fatigue, and other health issues....

In this comprehensive guide, "Metabolism Mastery: Breaking Free from Sabotaging Habits," we will delve deep into the world of metabolism. Each chapter will provide you with valuable insights and practical tips to optimize your metabolism, enhance your energy levels, and achieve your health goals....

Chapter 1: The Importance of Metabolism...

Metabolism is the sum of all chemical reactions within the body that sustain life. It's responsible for converting the food we eat into energy, repairing tissues, and removing waste products. Understanding its significance is the first step in taking control of your health....

Metabolism isn't just about weight management; it affects every aspect of your well-being. A well-functioning metabolism can help you maintain a healthy weight, support your immune system, and improve your mood....

The Metabolic Rate...

Your metabolic rate, often referred to as your metabolism, determines how quickly your body burns calories. It's influenced by various factors, including genetics, age, gender, and muscle mass. By understanding these factors, you can tailor your lifestyle to boost your metabolic rate....

Metabolism and Weight Management...

One of the most common misconceptions is that weight gain or loss is solely determined by calorie intake. While calories matter, metabolism plays a significant role. A sluggish metabolism can make it challenging to shed unwanted pounds, even with a reduced-calorie diet....

Metabolism and Energy...

Have you ever wondered why some people seem to have boundless energy while others struggle to get through the day? Metabolism holds the key. Optimizing your metabolism can provide you with the vitality needed to excel in all areas of your life....

Metabolism and Aging...

As we age, our metabolism naturally slows down. However, lifestyle choices can either exacerbate this decline or mitigate its effects. Chapter 14 will delve deeper into strategies for maintaining a youthful metabolism....

In the chapters that follow, we'll explore the various factors that influence metabolism, from dietary choices to exercise routines, sleep patterns, and even stress management. Armed with this knowledge, you'll be better equipped to make informed decisions and break free from habits that may be sabotaging your metabolism. It's time to embark on a journey to metabolic mastery, where you take charge of your health and vitality....

Chapter 2: Eating Habits and Their Impact on Metabolism...

In Chapter 1, we established the fundamental importance of metabolism in our daily lives. Now, let's dive into one of the most critical aspects of metabolism: our eating habits. What and how we eat can either fuel our metabolic fire or douse it with cold water....

The Role of Nutrients...

The food we consume provides our bodies with essential nutrients, including carbohydrates, proteins, fats, vitamins, and minerals. These nutrients are the building blocks and fuel for our metabolism. Understanding how to balance them is crucial for metabolic health....

Carbohydrates: The Energy Source...

Carbohydrates are your body's primary source of energy. Complex carbohydrates found in whole grains, fruits, and vegetables provide sustained energy, while simple carbohydrates like sugars offer quick but short-lived bursts....

Proteins: Building and Repair...

Proteins are essential for tissue repair and muscle building. They also play a role in various metabolic processes. Including lean protein sources like poultry, fish, and legumes in your diet is essential....

Fats: The Good and the Bad...

Not all fats are created equal. While some fats are healthy and necessary for metabolic functions, others can be detrimental. Understanding the difference between healthy fats (found in avocados, nuts, and olive oil) and unhealthy fats (found in processed foods) is key....

Meal Timing and Frequency...

When and how often you eat can influence your metabolic rate. Skipping meals or going too long without food can slow down metabolism and lead to overeating later in the day. On the other hand, eating balanced meals at regular intervals can help keep your metabolism revved up....

Metabolism-Boosting Foods...

Certain foods have been shown to have a thermogenic effect, meaning they temporarily boost your metabolic rate. These include spicy foods, green tea, and foods high in fiber. Incorporating these into your diet can give your metabolism a little extra kick....

Hydration and Metabolism...

Staying well-hydrated is essential for metabolic efficiency. Even mild dehydration can slow down your metabolism. Make sure to drink plenty of water throughout the day....

Mindful Eating...

Eating mindfully involves paying attention to what you eat, savoring each bite, and recognizing when you're full. This practice can prevent overeating and promote healthy digestion, both of which are essential for optimal metabolism....

In this chapter, we've scratched the surface of the intricate relationship between your eating habits and metabolism. As we progress through the book, you'll gain a deeper understanding of how to fine-tune your diet to support a healthy and efficient metabolism. Remember, each chapter is a building block towards metabolic mastery, and it's time to take the first step towards a healthier you....

Chapter 3: The Role of Physical Activity in Boosting Metabolism...

In Chapter 2, we explored the significance of our dietary choices in influencing metabolism. Now, let's turn our attention to another vital aspect of metabolism: physical activity. Exercise is not only essential for overall health but also a powerful tool for enhancing your metabolic rate....

Understanding Exercise and Metabolism...

Exercise triggers a series of metabolic responses that have far-reaching benefits. Here's how physical activity influences metabolism:...

Muscle Mass Matters...

One of the most significant factors contributing to your metabolic rate is your muscle mass. Muscle tissue burns more calories at rest than fat tissue. Engaging in strength training and resistance exercises can help you build and maintain lean muscle mass, thereby increasing your metabolic rate....

Cardiovascular Exercise...

Aerobic or cardiovascular exercise, such as running, swimming, or cycling, not only burns calories during the activity but also elevates your metabolic rate even after you've finished exercising. This phenomenon is known as the "afterburn" effect or excess post-exercise oxygen consumption (EPOC)....

Hormones and Exercise...

Physical activity influences the release of hormones like adrenaline and cortisol, which can affect your metabolism. Regular exercise helps regulate these hormones, reducing stress and supporting metabolic balance....

Age and Exercise...

As mentioned in the introduction, metabolism naturally slows down with age. However, regular physical activity can help mitigate this decline. It's never too late to start incorporating exercise into your routine....

Finding the Right Exercise Routine...

The type and intensity of exercise that work best for you may vary depending on your fitness level, goals, and preferences. Whether it's a brisk walk, a yoga class, or high-intensity interval training (HIIT), the key is to find an activity you enjoy and can sustain over the long term....

Combining Diet and Exercise...

For optimal metabolic health, it's essential to strike a balance between your diet and exercise routine. Properly fueling your body with the right nutrients before and after exercise can maximize its benefits....

Breaking Down Barriers...

Many people face barriers to regular exercise, such as time constraints, physical limitations, or lack of motivation. In this chapter, we'll address these challenges and provide practical tips for overcoming them....

Remember, improving your metabolic rate through physical activity is not just about weight management; it's about enhancing your overall well-being. In the subsequent chapters, we'll continue to explore various aspects of metabolism and provide you with actionable strategies for breaking free from sabotaging habits. So, lace up your sneakers and get ready to boost your metabolism through the power of movement....

Chapter 4: Sleep and Stress - Unseen Factors Affecting Metabolism...

In our exploration of metabolism, we've covered the importance of diet and exercise. Now, let's shed light on two often overlooked but significant factors: sleep and stress. These invisible influencers play a substantial role in determining the efficiency of your metabolism....

The Sleep-Metabolism Connection...

Sleep is a fundamental biological process that allows your body to rest, repair, and rejuvenate. But did you know that it also has a profound impact on your metabolism?...

Sleep Duration...

Getting an adequate amount of quality sleep is essential for metabolic health. Chronic sleep deprivation disrupts the hormonal balance responsible for appetite regulation, often leading to overeating and weight gain....

Circadian Rhythms...

Your body operates on a 24-hour internal clock known as the circadian rhythm. Disruptions to this rhythm, such as irregular sleep patterns or night-shift work, can negatively affect metabolism and increase the risk of metabolic disorders....

Sleep Disorders...

Conditions like sleep apnea and insomnia can interfere with your ability to achieve restorative sleep. Addressing these disorders is crucial for supporting metabolic balance....

The Stress-Metabolism Connection...

Stress is an inevitable part of life, but chronic stress can wreak havoc on your metabolism. Here's how stress affects your metabolic health:...

Hormonal Impact...

When you're stressed, your body releases hormones like cortisol and adrenaline. While these hormones are essential for the fight-or-flight response, prolonged elevation can disrupt metabolic processes and lead to weight gain, particularly around the abdominal area....

Emotional Eating...

Stress often triggers emotional eating, where individuals turn to comfort foods high in sugar and fat. These choices can have a detrimental impact on metabolic health....

Coping Mechanisms...

Learning effective stress management techniques, such as mindfulness, meditation, or exercise, can help mitigate the negative effects of chronic stress on metabolism....

The Importance of Balance...

Achieving balance in both sleep and stress management is essential for maintaining a healthy metabolism. In this chapter, we'll delve into strategies for improving sleep quality and managing stress effectively....

Holistic Wellness...

Remember, metabolism is not just about numbers on a scale; it's about overall wellness. By addressing these often underestimated factors, you can make significant strides toward optimizing your metabolic rate and achieving a healthier, more balanced life....

As we continue our journey through the intricacies of metabolism, keep in mind that each chapter builds upon the previous one, offering you a holistic approach to mastering your metabolism. Now, let's explore how hydration influences your metabolic health in Chapter 5....

Chapter 5: Hydration and Its Influence on Metabolism...

Hydration, often overlooked in the context of metabolism, plays a critical role in maintaining your body's optimal metabolic functions. In this chapter, we'll dive into the importance of staying well-hydrated and how it impacts your metabolism....

The Significance of Hydration...

Water is the essence of life, and your body is composed of about 60% water. Every cellular process, including those related to metabolism, relies on proper hydration....

Metabolic Processes...

Water is involved in nearly every metabolic reaction in your body. It helps transport nutrients, remove waste products, and regulate temperature....

Dehydration and Metabolism...

Even mild dehydration can slow down your metabolic rate. When you're dehydrated, your body's ability to burn calories efficiently is compromised....

Appetite Regulation...

Sometimes, thirst is mistaken for hunger. Staying adequately hydrated can prevent unnecessary snacking and overeating, which can negatively impact your metabolism....

How Much Water Do You Need?...

The amount of water you require can vary depending on factors like climate, activity level, and individual differences. As a general guideline, aim to drink at least eight 8-ounce glasses of water per day (the "8x8" rule). However, listen to your body; it's an excellent indicator of your hydration status....

Signs of Dehydration...

Recognizing the signs of dehydration is crucial. These can include dark urine, dry mouth, fatigue, and headaches. If you experience these symptoms, it's essential to increase your fluid intake....

Beyond Water...

While water is the primary source of hydration, you can also get fluids from foods like fruits and vegetables, as well as beverages like herbal tea and milk. Be mindful of your overall fluid intake....

Hydration Strategies...

In this chapter, we'll explore strategies for staying well-hydrated throughout the day, including practical tips for incorporating more fluids into your routine....

Remember, optimizing your metabolism is not just about diet and exercise; it's about nurturing your body's internal processes. By paying attention to your hydration needs and making conscious efforts to stay hydrated, you'll be taking another significant step toward metabolic mastery. In Chapter 6, we'll delve into the concept of nutrient timing and how it can impact your metabolism....

Chapter 6: The Power of Nutrient Timing...

Nutrient timing is a fascinating aspect of metabolism that revolves around when you consume specific nutrients. In this chapter, we'll explore how the timing of your meals and snacks can influence your metabolic rate and overall health....

Understanding Nutrient Timing...

Nutrient timing isn't just about what you eat; it's also about when you eat. The concept revolves around optimizing the delivery of nutrients to your body when it needs them most....

Pre-Workout Nutrition...

Eating a balanced meal or snack before exercise provides your body with the energy it needs to perform optimally. Carbohydrates, in particular, are essential for fueling your workouts....

Post-Workout Recovery...

After exercise, your body is in a prime state to absorb nutrients and repair muscle tissue. Protein and carbohydrates play a crucial role in post-workout recovery....

Meal Frequency...

The frequency of your meals and snacks throughout the day can impact your metabolism. Eating smaller, balanced meals every few hours can help maintain stable blood sugar levels and keep your metabolism revved up....

Nighttime Eating...

Eating late at night, especially heavy or high-calorie meals, can disrupt your sleep patterns and slow down your metabolism. It's essential to be mindful of what and when you eat in the evening....

Balancing Macronutrients...

Incorporating a balance of carbohydrates, proteins, and healthy fats into your meals and snacks is key to supporting your metabolism. We'll delve into the ideal macronutrient ratios for different times of the day....

Intermittent Fasting...

Intermittent fasting is an eating pattern that involves cycling between periods of fasting and eating. While it's not suitable for everyone, it can offer metabolic benefits when done correctly....

Personalizing Nutrient Timing...

Nutrient timing isn't one-size-fits-all. Your individual goals, activity level, and lifestyle play a significant role in determining the best timing for your meals and snacks. In this chapter, we'll help you tailor nutrient timing to your unique needs....

By mastering the art of nutrient timing, you can optimize your metabolism, improve your workout performance, and enhance your overall well-being. As we continue our journey through metabolic mastery, keep in mind that each chapter builds upon the previous one, offering you a comprehensive guide to breaking free from sabotaging habits. In Chapter 7, we'll explore the world of superfoods and their impact on metabolic health....

Chapter 7: Superfoods for Metabolic Health...

Superfoods are nutrient-dense foods that are packed with

vitamins, minerals, antioxidants, and other beneficial compounds. In this chapter, we'll explore the world of superfoods and how they can positively impact your metabolic health....

What Are Superfoods?...

Superfoods are not just a marketing buzzword; they are real foods that offer exceptional nutritional value. They can support your metabolism in various ways:...

Antioxidant Power...

Many superfoods are rich in antioxidants, which help combat oxidative stress and inflammation in the body. Reduced inflammation can contribute to a more efficient metabolism....

Nutrient Density...

Superfoods are nutrient powerhouses, meaning they provide a high concentration of essential vitamins and minerals for relatively few calories. This nutrient density supports overall health and metabolic function....

Fiber Content...

Fiber is essential for digestive health and can help regulate blood sugar levels. Some superfoods are excellent sources of dietary fiber, promoting a stable metabolism....

A Look at Superfoods...

We'll explore some popular superfoods and their specific benefits for metabolic health:...

Berries: Blueberries, strawberries, and other berries are rich in antioxidants and fiber, supporting both metabolism and heart health....

Leafy Greens: Spinach, kale, and other leafy greens are packed with vitamins, minerals, and fiber, promoting a healthy metabolism....

Nuts and Seeds: Almonds, chia seeds, and flaxseeds are nutrient-dense sources of healthy fats, protein, and fiber....

Fatty Fish: Salmon, mackerel, and sardines are high in omega-3 fatty acids, which can reduce inflammation and support metabolic function....

Green Tea: Green tea contains antioxidants called catechins, which have been shown to boost metabolism and aid in weight loss....

Incorporating Superfoods...

We'll provide practical tips on how to incorporate superfoods into your daily diet, making it easy to reap their metabolic benefits....

Variety and Balance...

While superfoods are beneficial, it's essential to maintain a balanced diet that includes a wide range of foods. A diverse diet ensures you get all the essential nutrients your body needs....

Supplements vs. Whole Foods...

We'll also discuss the pros and cons of using superfood supplements versus consuming these foods in their whole form....

By adding superfoods to your diet, you can enhance your metabolic health, support weight management, and improve your overall well-being. As we continue our journey through metabolic mastery, remember that each chapter builds upon the previous one, offering you a comprehensive guide to breaking free from sabotaging habits. In Chapter 8, we'll explore the impact of aging on metabolism and strategies to maintain a youthful metabolism....

Chapter 8: Metabolism and Aging - What You Need to Know...

Aging is an inevitable part of life, and as we grow older, our metabolism naturally undergoes changes. In this chapter, we'll explore the impact of aging on metabolism and provide strategies to maintain a youthful and efficient metabolism....

Metabolic Changes with Age...

As we age, several factors contribute to changes in our metabolic rate:...

Muscle Mass Reduction...

One of the most significant contributors to a declining metabolism is the gradual loss of muscle mass, known as sarcopenia. Muscle tissue burns more calories at rest than fat tissue, so a reduction in muscle mass can slow down metabolism....

Hormonal Shifts...

Hormonal changes, such as a decrease in growth hormone and sex hormones like estrogen and testosterone, can affect metabolism. These changes can lead to increased fat storage and decreased muscle mass....

Decreased Physical Activity...

Many individuals become less physically active as they age, which can further contribute to muscle loss and a slower metabolism....

Basal Metabolic Rate (BMR) Decline...

BMR, the number of calories your body needs at rest, tends to decrease with age. This means that as you get older, you may require fewer calories to maintain your weight....

Strategies for Maintaining a Youthful Metabolism...

While you can't stop the aging process, you can take steps to mitigate its effects on your metabolism:...

Strength Training...

Engaging in regular strength training exercises can help counteract muscle loss and boost your metabolism....

Cardiovascular Exercise...

Aerobic exercises like walking, jogging, or swimming can help maintain cardiovascular health and support a healthy metabolism....

Balanced Diet...

Eating a well-balanced diet that includes lean proteins, whole grains, fruits, vegetables, and healthy fats is essential for supporting metabolism as you age....

Hormone Replacement Therapy...

In some cases, hormone replacement therapy (HRT) may be recommended to address hormonal imbalances associated with aging. Consult with a healthcare professional for guidance....

Stress Management...

Chronic stress can accelerate the aging process and negatively impact metabolism. Incorporate stress-reduction techniques like meditation and yoga into your routine....

Embracing the Aging Process...

It's important to remember that aging is a natural part of life, and maintaining a youthful metabolism doesn't mean trying to turn back the clock. Instead, it's about embracing the wisdom and experiences that come with age while prioritizing your health and well-being....

In this chapter, we've explored how aging affects metabolism and provided strategies to support a vibrant and energetic life as you grow older. As we continue our journey through metabolic mastery, each chapter builds upon the previous one, offering you a comprehensive guide to breaking free from sabotaging habits. In Chapter 9, we'll delve into the intricate relationship between hormones and metabolism....

Chapter 9: Hormones and Metabolism - Balancing the Scales...

Hormones are the body's messengers, orchestrating various metabolic processes. In this chapter, we'll explore the intricate relationship between hormones and metabolism, and how you can balance the scales for optimal metabolic health....

The Hormonal Orchestra...

Hormones play a pivotal role in regulating metabolism. Here are some key hormones and their metabolic functions:...

Insulin...

Insulin is produced by the pancreas and is essential for regulating blood sugar levels. It helps transport glucose into cells for energy or storage....

Thyroid Hormones...

Thyroid hormones, including thyroxine (T4) and

triiodothyronine (T3), control your basal metabolic rate (BMR). An imbalance in thyroid hormones can lead to metabolic disturbances....

Leptin and Ghrelin...

These hormones regulate hunger and appetite. Leptin signals fullness, while ghrelin signals hunger. An imbalance can lead to overeating and weight gain....

Cortisol...

Cortisol, the stress hormone, can affect metabolism by influencing glucose metabolism and fat storage. Chronic stress can lead to cortisol imbalances....

Sex Hormones...

Estrogen and testosterone play roles in metabolism. Changes in these hormones, particularly during menopause or andropause, can impact body composition and metabolism....

Balancing Hormones for Metabolic Health...

Maintaining hormonal balance is crucial for metabolic health. Here are some strategies to achieve this balance:...

Diet and Nutrient Quality...

Eating a balanced diet that includes a variety of nutrients can support hormonal balance. For example, consuming omega-3 fatty acids can help reduce inflammation and improve insulin sensitivity....

Stress Management...

Chronic stress can disrupt hormonal balance. Incorporate stress-reduction techniques into your daily routine to support metabolic health....

Regular Physical Activity...

Exercise can help regulate hormones, including insulin and cortisol. Both aerobic and strength training exercises are beneficial....

Sleep Hygiene...

Prioritize good sleep habits, as sleep plays a vital role in hormone regulation. Aim for 7-9 hours of quality sleep per night....

Hormone Replacement Therapy (HRT)...

In some cases, hormonal imbalances may require medical intervention, such as hormone replacement therapy. Consult with a healthcare professional for guidance....

Individualized Approach...

Remember that hormonal balance is highly individualized. What works for one person may not work for another. It's essential to listen to your body and seek professional guidance when needed....

By understanding the role of hormones in metabolism and taking steps to balance them, you can optimize your metabolic health and overall well-being. As we continue our journey through metabolic mastery, each chapter builds upon the previous one, offering you a comprehensive guide to breaking free from sabotaging habits. In Chapter 10, we'll explore the concept of mindful eating and how it can transform your relationship with food and metabolism....

Chapter 10: Mindful Eating for a Revved-Up Metabolism...

In a world filled with distractions and fast-paced living, mindful eating offers a powerful approach to transform your relationship with food and boost your metabolism. In this chapter, we'll explore the concept of mindful eating and how it can positively impact your metabolic health....

What is Mindful Eating?...

Mindful eating is a practice that involves paying full attention to the present moment while eating. It's about savoring each bite, tuning into your body's hunger and fullness cues, and cultivating a deeper connection with the food you consume....

Benefits of Mindful Eating...

Improved Digestion: Mindful eating promotes better digestion by allowing your body to fully process and absorb nutrients....

Enhanced Satisfaction: By savoring each bite, you'll find

greater satisfaction in your meals, reducing the urge to overeat....

Weight Management: Mindful eating can support weight loss or maintenance by helping you make conscious, healthful choices....

Stress Reduction: This practice can reduce stress-related eating and emotional eating, which can negatively impact metabolism....

How to Practice Mindful Eating...

Here are some practical steps to incorporate mindful eating into your daily life:...

Slow Down...

Eat at a slower pace, taking the time to chew your food thoroughly. This allows your body to send signals of fullness to your brain....

Eliminate Distractions...

Turn off the TV, put away your phone, and create a calm eating environment. Minimize distractions to fully focus on your meal....

Engage Your Senses...

Take a moment to appreciate the colors, textures, and aromas of your food. Engage all your senses in the eating experience....

Listen to Your Body...

Pay attention to hunger and fullness cues. Eat when you're hungry and stop when you're satisfied, not overly full....

Practice Gratitude...

Express gratitude for the nourishment your food provides. Cultivating a positive mindset around eating can promote healthier choices....

Mindful Portion Control...

Be mindful of portion sizes, and use smaller plates to help control portions without feeling deprived....

The Metabolic Connection...

Mindful eating can positively influence metabolism in several ways:...

Better Digestion...

By thoroughly chewing your food and eating slowly, you support efficient digestion and nutrient absorption....

Reduced Stress...

Mindful eating can reduce stress-related eating, preventing the release of stress hormones that can negatively affect metabolism....

Balanced Blood Sugar...

Being attuned to your body's hunger and fullness cues can help regulate blood sugar levels and prevent energy crashes....

A Lifelong Practice...

Mindful eating is not a diet but a lifelong practice that can transform your relationship with food and metabolism. It encourages a more intuitive and balanced approach to eating, aligning with the principles of metabolic mastery....

As we continue our journey through this comprehensive guide to breaking free from sabotaging habits, remember that each chapter builds upon the previous one. In Chapter 11, we'll explore the importance of building lean muscle mass for metabolic efficiency, shedding light on the powerful role of strength training in your metabolic journey....

Chapter 11: Building Lean Muscle Mass for Metabolic Efficiency...

In the quest for metabolic mastery, building lean muscle mass emerges as a powerful tool. In this chapter, we'll explore the significance of muscle in your metabolism and how incorporating strength training can rev up your metabolic efficiency....

The Muscle-Metabolism Connection...

Lean muscle mass is metabolically active tissue, meaning it burns calories even at rest. Here's how muscle impacts your metabolism:...

Increased Resting Metabolic Rate (RMR)...

RMR is the number of calories your body burns while at rest. Muscle tissue requires more energy to maintain than fat tissue, so having more muscle increases your RMR....

Improved Insulin Sensitivity...

Muscle plays a crucial role in regulating blood sugar. Building and maintaining muscle can enhance insulin sensitivity, reducing the risk of insulin resistance and type 2 diabetes....

Enhanced Fat Burning...

Muscle tissue is a primary site for fat oxidation. As you build muscle, your body becomes more efficient at burning stored fat for energy....

Post-Exercise Calorie Burn...

Strength training workouts create a metabolic "afterburn" effect, where your body continues to burn calories even after the workout is over....

The Benefits of Strength
Training...

Strength training, also known as
resistance training or
weightlifting, offers numerous
benefits for both metabolic health
and overall well-being:...

Muscle Building...

Strength training stimulates
muscle growth, helping you
increase your lean muscle mass....

Fat Loss...

As you build muscle, your body
becomes more efficient at burning
fat, contributing to weight loss or
maintenance....

Bone Health...

Strength training also promotes bone density, reducing the risk of osteoporosis....

Improved Metabolic Profile...

Regular strength training can lead to improvements in blood sugar levels, cholesterol levels, and blood pressure....

Enhanced Functional Fitness...

Strong muscles support better posture, balance, and overall physical function....

Getting Started with Strength Training...

If you're new to strength training, it's essential to start gradually and seek guidance from a fitness professional or trainer. Here are some tips to get started:...

Choose a variety of exercises that target different muscle groups....

Focus on proper form and technique to prevent injury....

Start with a weight that challenges you but allows you to complete a set with good form....

Gradually increase the weight and intensity of your workouts over time....

Incorporating Strength Training into Your Routine...

To maximize the metabolic benefits of strength training, aim for at least two to three sessions per week. You can choose to work with free weights, resistance bands, or machines, depending on your preferences and access to equipment....

As we continue our journey toward metabolic mastery, remember that each chapter builds upon the previous one. In Chapter 12, we'll explore the impact of genetics on metabolism and how understanding your genetic predispositions can empower your health choices....

Chapter 12: The Impact of Genetics on Metabolism...

Genetics play a significant role in shaping your metabolism and overall health. In this chapter, we'll explore how your genetic makeup influences various aspects of metabolism and how understanding your genetic predispositions can empower your health choices....

The Genetic Blueprint...

Your genes provide the blueprint for your body's metabolic processes. They influence how your body processes nutrients, regulates hormones, and responds to various lifestyle factors....

Metabolic Rate...

Genetics can determine your baseline metabolic rate, which is the number of calories your body burns at rest. Some individuals naturally have a faster metabolism, while others have a slower one....

Nutrient Metabolism...

Your genes influence how your body metabolizes carbohydrates, fats, and proteins. Some people may be more efficient at processing certain nutrients than others....

Hormone Regulation...

Genetics also play a role in how your body regulates hormones like insulin, cortisol, and thyroid hormones. Variations in these genes can impact your metabolic health....

Personalized Nutrition and Fitness...

Understanding your genetic predispositions can help you make more informed choices about your diet and exercise routine:...

Nutritional Needs...

Genetic testing can reveal insights into how your body responds to different diets. For example, some individuals may do better with a higher-carb, lower-fat diet, while others thrive on a higher-fat, lower-carb approach....

Exercise Response...

Genetics can also shed light on how your body responds to different types of exercise. It can help you tailor your fitness routine to optimize results....

Disease Risk...

Certain genetic variations can increase your risk of specific health conditions, such as obesity, diabetes, or heart disease. Knowing your genetic risk factors can motivate you to take preventive measures....

The Role of Epigenetics...

While your genetic code is relatively fixed, epigenetics refers to changes in gene expression that can be influenced by environmental factors. This means that lifestyle choices, such as diet, exercise, and stress management, can impact how your genes are expressed....

Genetic Testing...

Genetic testing, often available through commercial services, can provide insights into your genetic predispositions. However, it's crucial to interpret these results in consultation with a healthcare professional or genetic counselor....

The Power of Personalization...

By understanding your genetic makeup and how it interacts with your lifestyle choices, you can personalize your approach to diet, exercise, and overall health. This empowers you to make choices that align with your genetic predispositions and can lead to better metabolic health....

As we continue our journey toward metabolic mastery,

remember that each chapter builds upon the previous one. In Chapter 13, we'll explore the world of supplements and their potential impact on metabolism, providing guidance on how to make informed choices in the realm of dietary supplements....

Chapter 13: The World of Supplements and Their Impact on Metabolism...

Dietary supplements have gained popularity as tools to enhance metabolic health and overall well-being. In this chapter, we'll explore the world of supplements, their potential impact on metabolism, and how to make informed choices when considering supplementation....

Understanding Dietary
Supplements...

Dietary supplements encompass a
wide range of products, including
vitamins, minerals, herbal extracts,
amino acids, and more. They are
designed to supplement your diet
with specific nutrients that may be
lacking or needed in higher
quantities....

Common Supplements for
Metabolism...

Several supplements are often
associated with metabolic
health:...

Vitamins: B vitamins, such as B12
and B6, play roles in energy
metabolism. Vitamin D is also
linked to metabolic function....

Minerals: Minerals like magnesium, zinc, and chromium are involved in various metabolic processes....

Omega-3 Fatty Acids: These essential fats have been shown to support metabolic health and reduce inflammation....

Protein Supplements: Protein powders can aid in muscle building and recovery, which can boost metabolism....

Herbal Extracts: Some herbal supplements, like green tea extract and cinnamon, have been studied for their potential metabolic benefits....

Considerations Before Supplementing...

Before adding supplements to your regimen, consider the following:...

Dietary Evaluation...

Assess your diet to identify any nutrient deficiencies. Supplements should complement a balanced diet, not replace it....

Individual Needs...

Supplement needs can vary based on age, gender, activity level, and specific health conditions. Consult with a healthcare professional or registered dietitian for personalized guidance....

Quality Matters...

Choose reputable brands and products. Look for third-party

testing and quality certifications to ensure product safety and efficacy....

Potential Interactions...

Be aware of potential interactions between supplements and medications you may be taking. Always consult with your healthcare provider if you have concerns....

Dosage and Timing...

Follow recommended dosages and guidelines for optimal results. Taking too much of certain supplements can have adverse effects....

Supplements and Metabolic Health...

While supplements can play a role in supporting metabolic health, they are not a substitute for a healthy diet and lifestyle. The foundation of metabolic mastery remains proper nutrition, regular exercise, stress management, and other lifestyle factors....

Holistic Approach...

The best approach to metabolic health is a holistic one that considers your overall well-being. Supplements should complement your efforts in maintaining a balanced and healthy lifestyle....

As we continue our journey toward metabolic mastery, remember that each chapter builds upon the previous one. In Chapter 14, we'll explore the impact of sleep and circadian rhythms on metabolism, shedding light on how prioritizing rest can be a powerful tool in optimizing your metabolic health....

Chapter 14: The Sleep-Metabolism Connection - Unlocking the Power of Rest...

In our fast-paced world, the importance of sleep is often underestimated. However, it plays a pivotal role in metabolic health and overall well-being. In this chapter, we'll delve into the intricate relationship between sleep and metabolism and how prioritizing rest can unlock the power of a healthier, more efficient metabolism....

The Vital Role of Sleep...

Sleep is a fundamental physiological process that allows your body to rest, recover, and rejuvenate. It's during sleep that your body performs essential functions that impact metabolism:...

Hormonal Regulation...

Sleep is crucial for hormonal balance. Insufficient sleep can disrupt hormones like insulin, cortisol, and ghrelin, leading to metabolic imbalances....

Cellular Repair...

During deep sleep, your body engages in repair and maintenance at the cellular level. This includes tissue repair, muscle growth, and immune system support....

Cognitive Function...

Quality sleep is essential for cognitive function, decision-making, and emotional well-being. Poor sleep can lead to stress, which in turn can negatively impact metabolism....

Sleep Duration and Metabolism...

The duration of your sleep matters when it comes to metabolic health:...

Appetite Regulation...

Lack of sleep can disrupt the hormones that regulate appetite, leading to increased hunger and cravings, often for high-calorie, sugary foods....

Blood Sugar Control...

Sleep deprivation can impair insulin sensitivity, making it harder for your body to regulate blood sugar levels. This can increase the risk of insulin resistance and type 2 diabetes....

Weight Management...

Poor sleep is associated with weight gain and obesity. It can affect your ability to lose weight and maintain a healthy body composition....

Improving Sleep Quality...

To harness the power of sleep for metabolic health, consider the following tips:...

Prioritize Sleep...

Make sleep a priority by setting a consistent sleep schedule and creating a relaxing bedtime routine....

Sleep Environment...

Create a comfortable sleep environment that is dark, quiet, and cool. Invest in a comfortable mattress and pillows....

Limit Screen Time...

Reduce exposure to screens (phones, tablets, TVs) before bedtime, as the blue light emitted can interfere with sleep....

Avoid Stimulants...

Limit caffeine and alcohol intake, especially in the hours leading up to bedtime....

Stress Management...

Practice stress-reduction techniques like meditation, deep breathing, or progressive muscle relaxation to calm your mind before sleep....

The Power of Circadian Rhythms...

Your body operates on a natural 24-hour internal clock known as the circadian rhythm. Disrupting this rhythm, such as with irregular sleep patterns or shift work, can negatively affect metabolism. It's essential to align your sleep-wake cycle with your body's natural rhythm....

A Holistic Approach...

Optimizing your metabolism is not just about diet and exercise; it's about nurturing your body's internal processes. Prioritizing quality sleep is a vital component of this holistic approach....

As we continue our journey toward metabolic mastery, remember that each chapter builds upon the previous one. In Chapter 15, our final chapter, we'll sum up the key takeaways and provide a roadmap for implementing lasting changes to achieve a healthier metabolism and overall well-being....

Chapter 15: Mastering Your Metabolism - A Roadmap to Lasting Change...

Congratulations on reaching the final chapter of our comprehensive guide to metabolic mastery! By now, you've gained a deep understanding of metabolism and the factors that influence it. In this concluding chapter, we'll sum up the key takeaways and provide you with a roadmap for implementing lasting changes to achieve a healthier metabolism and overall well-being....

Recap of Key Takeaways...

Let's briefly recap the essential points covered in this journey:...

Awareness: Recognize the role of metabolism in your overall health and well-being. Understand that it's a complex interplay of factors, not just about weight....

Nutrition: A balanced diet that includes a variety of nutrients is fundamental to a healthy metabolism. Focus on whole foods, lean proteins, fiber, and nutrient-dense choices....

Exercise: Regular physical activity, including both cardiovascular and strength training exercises, supports metabolic efficiency, muscle growth, and fat loss....

Sleep: Prioritize sleep and create a conducive sleep environment to support hormonal balance, appetite regulation, and overall metabolic health....

Stress Management: Chronic stress can disrupt metabolism. Incorporate stress-reduction techniques like meditation, mindfulness, or yoga into your routine....

Hydration: Staying well-hydrated is essential for efficient metabolic processes. Follow the "8x8" rule as a general guideline....

Nutrient Timing: Understand when and what you eat matters. Pre- and post-workout nutrition, meal frequency, and mindful eating can positively impact metabolism....

Superfoods: Incorporate nutrient-dense superfoods into your diet to provide essential vitamins, minerals, and antioxidants that support metabolic health....

Aging: Recognize the natural changes in metabolism that come with aging. Focus on maintaining muscle mass, hormonal balance, and overall well-being....

Hormones: Hormones play a significant role in metabolism. Balance insulin, cortisol, thyroid hormones, and sex hormones for optimal metabolic health....

Genetics: Your genetic makeup influences metabolism. Understanding your genetic predispositions can guide personalized nutrition and fitness choices....

Supplements: While supplements can support metabolic health, they should complement a balanced diet and lifestyle. Consult with a healthcare professional for guidance....

Mindful Eating: Practice mindful eating to savor your meals, tune into hunger cues, and build a positive relationship with food....

Your Roadmap to Metabolic Mastery...

Now that you have a comprehensive understanding of metabolism, here's a roadmap to help you implement lasting changes:...

Assessment: Start by assessing your current habits and lifestyle. Identify areas where you can make improvements....

Goal Setting: Set specific, measurable, and realistic goals for your metabolic health. These goals may include weight management, blood sugar control, or improved energy levels....

Plan of Action: Develop a personalized plan of action that incorporates the key principles discussed in this guide. Consider your dietary choices, exercise routine, sleep habits, and stress management techniques....

Consistency: Consistency is key to lasting change. Commit to your plan and make it a part of your daily life....

Monitoring: Keep track of your progress. Use tools like a food journal, fitness tracker, or sleep diary to monitor your habits and assess your improvements....

Adaptability: Be flexible and willing to adjust your plan as needed. Life is dynamic, and your metabolic needs may change over time....

Seek Support: Don't hesitate to seek support from healthcare professionals, registered dietitians, personal trainers, or support groups. They can provide guidance, motivation, and accountability....

Mindfulness: Incorporate mindfulness into your daily routine, not just in eating but in all aspects of life. Cultivate awareness and presence....

Long-Term Perspective: Remember that metabolic mastery is a lifelong journey. Focus on sustainable changes that promote long-term health and well-being....

Celebrate Success: Celebrate your achievements, no matter how small. Recognize that every positive step you take is a win on your journey to metabolic mastery....

With this roadmap in hand, you have the tools and knowledge to take control of your metabolism and transform your health. Thank you for embarking on this journey with us. May your path to metabolic mastery be filled with vitality, wellness, and lasting positive change....